Breath Again

A Comprehensive Guide for Lung Cancer Patients

Olivia Freedman

Table of contents

INTRODUCTION

PART I

Treatment Options

PART II:

Managing the Physical Challenges of Lung Cancer

PART III

Navigating the Healthcare System

PART IV

Living with Lung Cancer

CONCLUSION

Moving Forward: Resources for Living with Lung Cancer

INTRODUCTION

Understanding Lung Cancer: Causes, Types, and Stages

Lung cancer is a complex and often misunderstood disease. It occurs when abnormal cells grow and multiplies uncontrollably in the lungs, forming a tumor. Lung cancer can be caused by a variety of factors, including exposure to carcinogens such as tobacco smoke, air pollution, and radon gas. In rare cases, genetic mutations may also play a role in the development of lung cancer.

There are two main types of lung cancer: non-small cell lung cancer (NSCLC) and small cell lung cancer (SCLC). NSCLC is the most common type of lung cancer and accounts for approximately 85% of all cases. SCLC, on the other hand, is less common and tends to grow more quickly than NSCLC.

Lung cancer is also classified by its stage, which describes the extent and severity of the disease. The stages of lung cancer range from Stage 0 (the earliest stage) to Stage IV (the most advanced stage). Stage 0 lung cancer is limited to the inner lining of the lung, while Stage IV lung cancer has spread to other parts of the body.

Understanding the causes, types, and stages of lung cancer is essential for patients and their loved ones as they navigate the complexities of the disease. By working closely with a team of medical professionals and staying informed about the latest research and treatment options, lung cancer patients can take an active role in managing their health and well-being.

Symptoms and Diagnosis: What to Expect
Symptoms of lung cancer can vary widely depending on the type and stage of the disease. Some common symptoms of lung cancer include

persistent cough, chest pain, shortness of breath, hoarseness, and coughing up blood. However, it's important to note that many people with lung cancer may not experience any symptoms in the early stages of the disease.

If you are experiencing symptoms that could be related to lung cancer, your doctor will likely perform a series of tests to diagnose the disease. These may include imaging tests such as X-rays, CT scans, or MRI scans, as well as a biopsy, in which a small sample of tissue is removed from the lung and analyzed for cancer cells.

The diagnosis of lung cancer can be a difficult and emotional experience for patients and their loved ones. It's important to remember that early detection and treatment can improve outcomes and increase the chances of survival. Working closely with a team of medical professionals, including oncologists, pulmonologists, and radiologists, can help ensure that you receive the best possible care and support throughout the diagnostic and treatment process.

If you have been diagnosed with lung cancer, it's important to stay informed about your treatment options and to seek out support from family, friends, and other resources. Many organizations and support groups exist to provide information and emotional support for those affected by lung cancer, and your healthcare team can help you connect with these resources as needed.

Coping with the Emotional Impact of Lung Cancer

Being diagnosed with lung cancer can be a highly emotional and challenging experience, both for patients and their loved ones. Coping with the emotional impact of the disease is an essential part of managing lung cancer and can help improve the quality of life for those affected.

Some common emotional responses to a lung cancer diagnosis may include fear, anxiety, depression, anger, and a sense of loss or grief. These emotions are normal and understandable given the seriousness of the disease, and it's important to recognize and acknowledge them.

There are several strategies that can help patients and their loved ones cope with the emotional impact of lung cancer. These may include:

1. Seeking out support: Talking to friends, family members, or a mental health professional can provide a valuable outlet for emotions and help patients and caregivers feel less isolated.

2. Practicing self-care: Engaging in activities that promote physical and emotional well-being, such as exercise, meditation, or hobbies, can help reduce stress and improve mood.

3. Staying informed: Staying up-to-date on the latest research and treatment options can help patients feel more empowered and in control of their health.

4. Finding meaning: Engaging in activities that provide a sense of purpose or meaning, such as volunteering or participating in support groups, can help patients and caregivers feel connected to something larger than themselves.

5. Planning for the future: Discussing end-of-life care and making plans for the future can help alleviate anxiety and provide a sense of control and comfort.

Coping with the emotional impact of lung cancer is an ongoing process, and patients and caregivers may need to revisit these strategies and seek out new sources of support over time. With the right resources and support, however, it is possible to manage the emotional challenges of lung cancer and maintain a sense of hope and resilience.

PART I

Treatment Options

Surgery, Radiation, and Chemotherapy: Pros and Cons

Surgery, radiation therapy, and chemotherapy are three of the most common treatments for lung cancer. Each of these approaches has its own pros and cons, and the best treatment plan for each patient will depend on a variety of factors, including the type and stage of cancer, the patient's overall health, and personal preferences.

Surgery:

Surgery involves the removal of the tumor and surrounding tissue from the lung. The main benefit of surgery is that it can often provide a complete cure for early-stage lung cancer. However, surgery may not be an option for patients with advanced lung cancer or those who are not healthy enough to undergo the procedure.

Pros:

- Can provide a complete cure for early-stage lung cancer
- May reduce the risk of cancer spreading to other parts of the body
- Can help alleviate symptoms such as shortness of breath and coughing

Cons:

- Can be a major surgery with risks of complications
- May require a long recovery time
- May not be an option for patients with advanced or widespread cancer

Radiation Therapy:

Radiation therapy involves the use of high-energy radiation to kill cancer cells. It can be used alone or in combination with other treatments such as chemotherapy.

Pros:

- Can be effective at killing cancer cells
- May be used to shrink tumors before surgery or to treat cancer that has spread to other parts of the body
- Can be delivered using external beam radiation or implanted radioactive sources

Cons:

- May cause side effects such as fatigue, skin irritation, and nausea
- May damage healthy tissue surrounding the tumor

- May not be an option for patients with certain types of lung cancer or those who have had radiation therapy in the past

Chemotherapy:

Chemotherapy involves the use of drugs to kill cancer cells. It can be administered orally or through injection and is often used in combination with other treatments such as surgery or radiation therapy.

Pros:

- Can be effective at killing cancer cells throughout the body
- Can be used to shrink tumors before surgery or to treat cancer that has spread to other parts of the body
- Can be administered in a variety of ways, including orally or through injection

Cons:

- May cause side effects such as nausea, hair loss, and fatigue
- May damage healthy cells as well as cancer cells
- May not be an option for patients with certain types of lung cancer or those who are not healthy enough to undergo treatment

In summary, surgery, radiation therapy, and chemotherapy are all important tools in the fight against lung cancer. Each approach has its own unique benefits and drawbacks, and the best treatment plan for each patient will depend on a variety of factors. By working closely with a team of medical professionals and staying informed about the latest research and treatment options, lung cancer patients can make informed decisions about their care and achieve the best possible outcomes.

Targeted Therapy and Immunotherapy: Emerging Treatments

Targeted therapy and immunotherapy are two emerging treatments for lung cancer that offer new hope for patients who have not responded to traditional treatments such as surgery, radiation therapy, and chemotherapy. These treatments are designed to specifically target cancer cells while sparing healthy cells, which can reduce the risk of side effects and improve outcomes.

Targeted Therapy:

Targeted therapy involves the use of drugs that target specific proteins or genes that are involved in the growth and spread of cancer cells. These drugs are designed to disrupt the signaling pathways that allow cancer cells to survive and proliferate and can be administered orally or through injection.

Pros:

- Can be highly effective at treating certain types of lung cancer, particularly those with specific genetic mutations
- Can have fewer side effects than traditional chemotherapy
- Can be administered on an outpatient basis

Cons:

- May only be effective for patients with specific genetic mutations
- May be expensive and not covered by all insurance plans
- May eventually become less effective as cancer cells develop new mutations

Immunotherapy:

Immunotherapy involves the use of drugs that stimulate the body's immune system to recognize and attack cancer cells. These drugs work by targeting proteins on the surface of cancer cells that prevent the immune system from recognizing them as foreign.

Pros:

- Can be effective at treating certain types of lung cancer, particularly those with high levels of a protein called PD-L1
- Can have fewer side effects than traditional chemotherapy
- Can provide long-lasting benefits, as the immune system can continue to recognize and attack cancer cells even after treatment is complete

Cons:

- May only be effective for patients with specific types of lung cancer or high levels of PD-L1

- May cause side effects such as fatigue, skin rash, and inflammation
- May be expensive and not covered by all insurance plans

In summary, targeted therapy and immunotherapy are two emerging treatments for lung cancer that offer new hope for patients who have not responded to traditional treatments. While these treatments have their own unique benefits and drawbacks, they represent an exciting development in the field of cancer research and offer new opportunities for patients to achieve better outcomes. By working closely with a team of medical professionals and staying informed about the latest research and treatment options, lung cancer patients can make informed decisions about their care and achieve the best possible outcomes.

Integrative Medicine and Complementary Therapies

Integrative medicine and complementary therapies are becoming increasingly popular among lung cancer patients as a way to manage symptoms and improve overall well-being. Integrative medicine combines conventional medical treatments with complementary therapies, such as acupuncture, massage, and meditation, to address the physical, emotional, and spiritual needs of the patient. These therapies can be used alongside traditional treatments to help manage side effects and improve quality of life.

Acupuncture:

Acupuncture is a traditional Chinese medicine practice that involves inserting thin needles into specific points on the body to relieve pain and other symptoms. Some studies have shown that acupuncture can help relieve pain, nausea, and other symptoms commonly experienced by lung cancer patients.

Massage:

Massage therapy involves manipulating the soft tissues of the body to relieve tension and promote relaxation. It can be used to help manage pain, reduce stress, and improve overall well-being. Some studies have shown that massage therapy can help relieve pain and anxiety in lung cancer patients.

Meditation:

Meditation involves focusing the mind on a specific object, sound, or phrase to promote relaxation and reduce stress. It can be practiced alone or with the guidance of a trained professional. Some studies have shown that meditation can help reduce anxiety and depression in lung cancer patients.

Other complementary therapies that may be helpful for lung cancer patients include yoga, tai chi, and aromatherapy. It is important for patients to work closely with their healthcare team to determine which therapies are appropriate for their specific needs and medical history.

In summary, integrative medicine and complementary therapies can be helpful for lung cancer patients in managing symptoms and improving overall well-being. These therapies can be used alongside traditional treatments to help patients achieve better outcomes and improve their quality of life. By working closely with their healthcare team and staying informed about the latest research and treatment options, patients can make informed decisions about their care and achieve the best possible outcomes.

PART II:

Managing the Physical Challenges of Lung Cancer

Side Effects of Treatment: How to Cope

Side effects are a common concern for lung cancer patients undergoing treatment, such as surgery, radiation therapy, chemotherapy, targeted therapy, or immunotherapy. While these treatments can be effective in treating cancer, they can also cause a range of side effects that can affect a patient's quality of life. It is important for patients to be aware of potential side effects and to work closely with their healthcare team to manage them effectively.

Common side effects of lung cancer treatment include:

- Fatigue
- Nausea and vomiting

- Loss of appetite
- Hair loss
- Skin changes
- Mouth sores
- Infection
- Difficulty swallowing
- Diarrhea
- Constipation
- Neuropathy
- Depression and anxiety

To help manage side effects, patients may be prescribed medications or other interventions, such as:

- Anti-nausea drugs
- Pain relievers
- Steroids
- Nutritional supplements
- Anti-anxiety medication
- Physical therapy

- Support groups or counseling

In addition to medical interventions, there are also lifestyle changes that patients can make to help manage side effects. These may include:

- Eating a balanced diet
- Getting regular exercise
- Getting enough rest and sleep
- Avoiding alcohol and tobacco
-Practicing stress-reducing activities, such as meditation or yoga
- Staying hydrated

It is important for patients to communicate openly with their healthcare team about any side effects they are experiencing, as they may be able to offer additional support or adjustments to the treatment plan. Patients should also follow their treatment plan closely and attend all scheduled appointments to ensure the best possible outcomes.

In summary, side effects are a common concern for lung cancer patients undergoing treatment, but there are many strategies available to manage them effectively. By working closely with their healthcare team and making necessary lifestyle changes, patients can improve their quality of life and achieve the best possible outcomes.

Nutrition and Exercise: Tips for Staying Healthy

Nutrition and exercise are important aspects of overall health and can play a significant role in helping lung cancer patients manage symptoms, side effects of treatment, and improve overall well-being. Proper nutrition and regular exercise can help patients maintain strength, manage weight, improve sleep, reduce stress, and boost their immune system.

Here are some tips for staying healthy through nutrition and exercise:

Nutrition:

- Eat a balanced diet that includes plenty of fruits and vegetables, lean proteins, whole grains, and healthy fats.
- Stay hydrated by drinking plenty of water and limiting sugary drinks and alcohol.
- Work with a registered dietitian to create a meal plan that meets your specific nutritional needs and takes into account any dietary restrictions or side effects from treatment.
- Avoid processed foods, fried foods, and foods high in sugar and sodium.
- Consider taking supplements if your diet is lacking in certain nutrients.

Exercise:

- Incorporate regular exercise into your routine, such as walking, swimming, or cycling. Aim for at least 30 minutes of moderate exercise most days of the week.

- Work with a physical therapist or exercise specialist to develop an exercise plan that is safe and appropriate for your specific needs and fitness level.

- Consider incorporating strength training to maintain muscle mass and bone density.

- Listen to your body and rest when needed. It is important to find a balance between pushing yourself and allowing your body time to recover.

- If you are experiencing pain or discomfort, talk to your healthcare team before starting or continuing an exercise routine.

By focusing on proper nutrition and regular exercise, lung cancer patients can improve their overall health and well-being, manage symptoms and side effects, and potentially improve treatment outcomes. Working with healthcare professionals, such as a registered dietitian and physical therapist, can help patients develop a plan that is safe and effective for their specific needs.

Pain Management: Options and Strategies

Pain is a common symptom for many lung cancer patients, and can be caused by cancer itself or by the treatments used to manage it, such as surgery, radiation therapy, chemotherapy, targeted therapy, or immunotherapy. Effective pain management is important to help patients maintain their quality of life, manage other symptoms, and improve overall well-being.

Here are some options and strategies for managing pain associated with lung cancer:

Medications:

- Over-the-counter pain relievers, such as acetaminophen or ibuprofen, may be helpful for mild pain.

- Prescription pain medications, such as opioids, may be necessary for moderate to severe pain. It is important to work closely with a healthcare provider to find the right medication and dose, and to monitor for potential side effects or addiction risks.

Interventional Procedures:

- Nerve blocks or epidural injections may be used to provide pain relief in specific areas of the body.

- Radiation therapy or ablation therapy may be used to target specific areas of pain caused by cancer.

Complementary Therapies:

- Acupuncture, massage therapy, or mindfulness practices may help reduce pain and improve overall well-being.
- Heat or cold therapy may provide relief for specific types of pain.

It is important for patients to work closely with their healthcare team to find the best pain management options for their specific needs. Patients should communicate openly about the location, type, and intensity of their pain, as well as any side effects or concerns they may have.

In addition to medical interventions, there are also lifestyle changes that may help manage pain, including:

- Getting enough rest and sleep
- Eating a balanced diet
- Getting regular exercise or physical therapy

- Practicing stress-reducing activities, such as meditation or yoga

By taking a comprehensive approach to pain management, lung cancer patients can improve their quality of life and maintain their overall well-being.

PART III

Navigating the Healthcare System

Finding the Right Medical Team: Questions to Ask

Finding the right medical team is crucial for lung cancer patients, as they will be working closely with healthcare professionals throughout their treatment journey. It is important to feel comfortable with the medical team and trust in their expertise and ability to provide the best possible care.

Here are some questions to consider when searching for the right medical team:

1. What are the credentials and experience of the medical team?
- Are they board-certified in their specialty?
- How many years of experience do they have in treating lung cancer patients?

- What is their success rate in treating lung cancer patients?

2. What are the treatment options available and what are the benefits and risks of each?
- What treatment options are available for the specific type and stage of lung cancer?
- What are the benefits and risks of each treatment option?
- What is the recommended treatment plan and why?

3. How will the medical team communicate with the patient and their family?
- How often will the medical team communicate with the patient and their family?
- Will there be a dedicated nurse or care coordinator who can answer questions and provide support?
- How can the patient and their family contact the medical team in case of an emergency or urgent need?

4. What supportive care services are available?

- Are there support groups or counseling services available to help cope with the emotional impact of lung cancer?

- Are there nutritionists, physical therapists, or other specialists available to help manage symptoms and side effects of treatment?

5. How will the medical team monitor the patient's progress?

- What tests or imaging will be used to monitor the patient's response to treatment?

- How often will these tests be conducted?

- How will the medical team adjust the treatment plan if necessary?

By asking these questions and discussing concerns with the medical team, lung cancer patients can feel more informed and empowered in their treatment decisions. It is important to find a medical team that is experienced, compassionate, and committed to providing the best possible care for each patient's individual needs.

Financial and Legal Considerations: Resources and Support

Dealing with a lung cancer diagnosis can be overwhelming, both emotionally and financially. It is important for patients and their families to be aware of the financial and legal considerations that may arise during the treatment process.

Here are some resources and support options for managing financial and legal considerations:

1. Health Insurance
- Understand your health insurance coverage and benefits, including deductibles, co-payments, and out-of-pocket maximums.

- Talk to your healthcare provider and insurance company about pre-authorization requirements for treatments and procedures.

2. Financial Assistance Programs
- Look into financial assistance programs, such as those offered by non-profit organizations, hospitals, and pharmaceutical companies.
- Contact government agencies, such as Medicare and Medicaid, to determine eligibility for financial assistance.

3. Legal Considerations
- Consider creating or updating legal documents, such as a will or power of attorney, to ensure that your wishes are respected.
- Talk to an attorney or financial planner about estate planning and tax implications.

4. Support Groups

- Join a support group or speak with a financial counselor to discuss strategies for managing financial stress and planning for the future.
- Connect with other patients and families who have gone through similar experiences.

5. Employee Assistance Programs (EAP)
- Ask your employer about EAP resources, which may provide financial counseling or legal advice to employees and their families.

By being proactive and seeking out resources and support, lung cancer patients and their families can better manage the financial and legal considerations that may arise during the treatment process. It is important to remember that there are resources available to help alleviate the financial burden and provide support during this challenging time.

Clinical Trials and Research: What You Need to Know

Clinical trials are research studies that investigate new treatments, diagnostic tools, or medical procedures to determine their safety and effectiveness. For lung cancer patients, clinical trials may offer the opportunity to receive cutting-edge treatments that are not yet widely available.

Here's what you need to know about clinical trials and research:

1. Clinical Trial Phases
- Clinical trials typically go through three phases before a new treatment is approved by the FDA for widespread use.
- Phase I trials are the first studies to test a new treatment in humans and are usually conducted with a small group of patients to evaluate safety and dosage.
- Phase II trials test the effectiveness of a treatment in a larger group of patients.

- Phase III trials compare the new treatment to standard treatments to determine which is more effective.

2. Eligibility
- Each clinical trial has specific eligibility criteria, such as age, gender, disease stage, and previous treatments.
- Talk to your healthcare provider about whether you might be eligible for a clinical trial.

3. Benefits and Risks
- Clinical trials offer the potential for access to new treatments that may be more effective than current treatments.
- However, there are also potential risks associated with clinical trials, such as side effects and uncertainty about the effectiveness of the treatment.

4. Informed Consent

- Before participating in a clinical trial, patients are required to provide informed consent, which means they have been informed of the risks and benefits of the study and understand what participation involves.
- Patients have the right to ask questions and receive information about the study before making a decision about whether to participate.

5. Finding Clinical Trials
- There are various resources available to help patients find clinical trials, such as the National Cancer Institute's Clinical Trials Search, ClinicalTrials.gov, and patient advocacy groups.
- Talk to your healthcare provider about whether participating in a clinical trial is a good option for you.

By understanding the basics of clinical trials and research, lung cancer patients can make informed decisions about their treatment options and potentially access new treatments that may improve their outcomes. It is important to discuss the potential benefits and risks with healthcare providers and loved ones before making a decision about whether to participate in a clinical trial.

PART IV

Living with Lung Cancer

Caregiving: Supporting a Loved One with Lung Cancer

Caring for a loved one with lung cancer can be a challenging and emotional experience. As a caregiver, it is important to provide support, both physically and emotionally, to ensure your loved one receives the best care possible. Here are some tips for supporting a loved one with lung cancer:

1. Communication
- Open and honest communication is essential. Ask your loved one how they are feeling and what you can do to help.
- Be a good listener and provide emotional support.

2. Assistance with Medical Care

- Help your loved one with scheduling appointments and transportation to and from appointments.
- Keep track of medications and ensure they are taken as prescribed.
- Help manage side effects of treatment, such as nausea or fatigue.

3. Practical Support
- Assist with daily tasks, such as cooking, cleaning, and running errands.
- Consider hiring a home health aide or personal care assistant to provide additional support.

4. Emotional Support
- Offer emotional support and be a good listener.
- Encourage your loved one to express their feelings and talk openly about their fears and concerns.
- Help your loved one stay connected to family and friends.

5. Self-Care

- Caring for a loved one can be emotionally and physically draining. It is important to take care of yourself as well.

- Make time for your own hobbies and interests.

- Seek support from other caregivers or a support group.

By providing support and being an advocate for your loved one, you can help them navigate the challenges of lung cancer treatment. Remember to take care of yourself and seek support when needed, as caregiving can be emotionally challenging.

Coping with Stress and Anxiety: Techniques for Self-Care

Being diagnosed with lung cancer can be a stressful and anxiety-provoking experience. Coping with stress and anxiety is important for maintaining overall physical and emotional well-being. Here are some techniques for self-care to help manage stress and anxiety:

1. Mindfulness
- Mindfulness techniques, such as deep breathing, meditation, or yoga, can help reduce stress and anxiety.
- Practice mindfulness regularly to build resilience and improve overall well-being.

2. Exercise
- Regular exercise can help improve mood and reduce stress levels.
- Even low-impact exercise, such as walking, can have a positive impact on mental health.

3. Social Support
- Stay connected with friends and family who provide emotional support and understanding.
- Join a support group or seek counseling to talk about your feelings and get additional support.

4. Relaxation Techniques
- Practice relaxation techniques, such as listening to calming music or taking a warm bath, to help reduce stress and anxiety.

5. Positive Thinking
- Try to focus on positive aspects of your life and your accomplishments.
- Set realistic goals and celebrate small successes along the way.

6. Self-Care Activities
- Take time for yourself and engage in activities that bring you joy, such as reading, cooking, or spending time outdoors.
- Make self-care a priority to help manage stress and anxiety.

By incorporating self-care techniques into your daily routine, you can better manage stress and anxiety related to lung cancer. Remember to seek support from loved ones or professional resources when needed, and be kind to yourself throughout the process. Coping with stress and anxiety is a journey, but with practice and persistence, it can become a manageable part of your overall lung cancer treatment plan.

Finding Hope and Inspiration: Stories of Survival and Resilience

When facing a lung cancer diagnosis, finding hope and inspiration can be a powerful tool for coping with the emotional and physical challenges of treatment. Here are some stories of survival and resilience to provide hope and inspiration during this difficult time:

1. Survivors' Stories

- Read or listen to stories of other individuals who have survived lung cancer to learn about their experiences and gain inspiration.

- Seek support groups or online communities where survivors share their stories and provide encouragement.

2. Celebrity Advocates
- Many celebrities and public figures have shared their experiences with lung cancer and become advocates for awareness and research.
- Learn about their stories and use their advocacy as a source of inspiration and hope.

3. Inspirational Quotes
- Search for inspirational quotes that can provide a sense of hope and positivity during difficult times.
- Write down or display these quotes in places where you will see them regularly, such as your workspace or on your phone.

4. Resilience Techniques
- Learn about resilience techniques, such as cognitive behavioral therapy or positive

psychology, to build your own resilience and find hope.
- Practice gratitude and mindfulness regularly to cultivate a positive outlook and sense of hope.

5. Art and Music
- Engage in art or music therapy to explore emotions and find inspiration.
- Create a playlist of music that brings you joy and listen to it regularly.

By finding sources of hope and inspiration, you can stay positive and resilient during the challenges of lung cancer treatment. Remember that everyone's journey is unique, and it is important to find what works best for you. Use these stories and techniques to find your own sense of hope and inspiration on your path to healing and recovery.

A Survival Story

Sarah was a 54-year-old woman who loved nothing more than spending time outdoors with her family. One day, she noticed a persistent cough and chest pain that just wouldn't go away. Concerned, she went to her doctor for a check-up.

After a series of tests, Sarah received the shocking news that she had Stage 3 lung cancer. She was devastated but determined to fight the disease with all her strength.

Sarah underwent surgery to remove the cancerous tumor, followed by several rounds of chemotherapy and radiation therapy. She experienced a range of side effects, including fatigue, hair loss, and difficulty sleeping, but remained focused on her goal of beating the disease.

Throughout her treatment, Sarah drew strength and inspiration from her family, who supported her every step of the way. They spent time together hiking, picnicking, and enjoying the beauty of nature, which helped Sarah stay positive and motivated.

After several months of treatment, Sarah received the wonderful news that she was in remission. Her lung cancer had been successfully treated, and she was able to resume her active lifestyle with her family.

Reflecting on her experience, Sarah was grateful for the medical professionals who had helped her through her treatment, as well as her family who provided her with endless love and support. She also felt empowered to share her story with others and advocate for lung cancer awareness and research.

Sarah's experience is a powerful reminder of the resilience of the human spirit, and the importance of hope and perseverance in the face of adversity.

CONCLUSION

Moving Forward: Resources for Living with Lung Cancer

Moving forward after a lung cancer diagnosis can be challenging, but there are many resources available to help individuals and their families cope with the disease and adjust to a new normal. Here are some resources to consider:

1. Support Groups
- Joining a support group can provide emotional support and a sense of community for individuals living with lung cancer and their loved ones.
- Groups can be found online or in person through organizations like the American Cancer Society or CancerCare.

2. Palliative Care

- Palliative care can provide relief from symptoms and improve the quality of life for individuals living with lung cancer.
- Palliative care specialists can work with medical teams to address physical and emotional needs and provide support for caregivers and families.

3. Rehabilitation Services
- Rehabilitation services, such as physical therapy or speech therapy, can help individuals with lung cancer regain strength and independence.
- Occupational therapy can help individuals with daily tasks and make adjustments to their home or work environment.

4. Financial Assistance
- Cancer treatment can be expensive, and financial assistance may be available to help cover costs.
- Resources like the American Cancer Society or Cancer Financial Assistance Coalition can provide

information on financial aid programs and resources.

5. Legal Assistance
- Individuals with lung cancer may face legal issues related to employment or insurance coverage.
- Legal aid organizations like Cancer Legal Resource Center can provide legal advice and support for individuals with lung cancer.

6. Survivorship Programs
- Survivorship programs provide resources and support for individuals who have completed treatment for lung cancer.
- Programs can offer guidance on managing long-term side effects, adjusting to life after treatment, and maintaining overall health and wellness.

By utilizing these resources, individuals with lung cancer and their loved ones can find the support and resources they need to move forward after a diagnosis. Remember, you are not alone and there are many people and organizations available to help you along the way.

Advocacy and Awareness: Making a Difference
Advocacy and awareness are essential components in the fight against lung cancer. By raising awareness of the disease and advocating for policies that support research and access to care, individuals and organizations can make a difference in the lives of those affected by lung cancer.

Here are some ways to get involved:

1. Join a Lung Cancer Advocacy Group
- Organizations like the Lung Cancer Research Foundation, LUNGevity Foundation, and American Lung Association offer opportunities to advocate for lung cancer research and policy changes.

2. Participate in Lung Cancer Walks and Events
- Lung cancer walks and events raise awareness and funds for research and support programs.
- Participating in these events can also provide an opportunity to connect with others affected by lung cancer.

3. Share Your Story
- Sharing personal experiences with lung cancer can help raise awareness and reduce the stigma surrounding the disease.
- Consider sharing your story through social media, blog posts, or other platforms.

4. Educate Yourself and Others
- Stay informed about the latest advances in lung cancer research and treatment options.
- Share this information with others to raise awareness and encourage others to get involved.

5. Advocate for Policy Changes

- Contact your elected officials to advocate for policies that support lung cancer research and access to care.
- Join campaigns and initiatives to support these efforts.

By becoming an advocate and raising awareness about lung cancer, individuals and organizations can make a significant impact in the fight against the disease. Together, we can work towards a future where lung cancer is no longer a leading cause of cancer-related deaths.

9 798392 187423